AF198660

Burn Fat – Reach Your Ideal Weight

Get Rid of Excess Fat and Get the Body of Your Dreams

Jamie Wolf

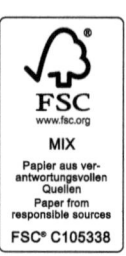

Bibliografische Information der Deutschen Nationalbibliothek:

Die Deutsche Nationalbibliothek verzeichnet diese Publikation in der Deutschen Nationalbibliografie; detaillierte bibliografische Daten sind im Internet über http://dnb.dnb.de abrufbar.

Herstellung und Verlag: BoD – Books on Demand, Norderstedt

ISBN: 978-3-7519-9514-6

Introduction

By using this book, you accept this disclaimer in full.

No advice

The book contains information. The information is not advice and should not be treated as such.

No representations or warranties

To the maximum extent permitted by applicable law and subject to section below, we exclude all representations, warranties, undertakings and guarantees relating to the book.

Without prejudice to the generality of the foregoing paragraph, we do not represent, warrant, undertake or guarantee:

- that the information in the book is correct, accurate, complete or non-misleading.

- that the use of the guidance in the book will lead to any particular outcome or result.

Limitations and exclusions of liability

The limitations and exclusions of liability set out in this section and elsewhere in this disclaimer: are subject to section 6 below; and govern all liabilities arising under the disclaimer or in relation to the book, including liabilities arising in contract, in tort (including negligence) and for breach of statutory duty.

We will not be liable to you in respect of any losses arising out of any event or events beyond our reasonable control.

We will not be liable to you in respect of any business losses, including without limitation loss of or damage to profits, income, revenue, use, production, anticipated savings, business, contracts, commercial opportunities or goodwill.

We will not be liable to you in respect of any loss or corruption of any data, database or software.

We will not be liable to you in respect of any special, indirect or consequential loss or damage.

Exceptions

Nothing in this disclaimer shall: limit or exclude our liability for death or personal injury resulting from negligence; limit or exclude our liability for fraud or fraudulent misrepresentation; limit any of our liabilities in any way that is not permitted under applicable law; or exclude any of our liabilities that may not be excluded under applicable law.

Severability

If a section of this disclaimer is determined by any court or other competent authority to be unlawful and/or unenforceable, the other sections of this disclaimer continue in effect.

If any unlawful and/or unenforceable section would be lawful or enforceable if part of it were deleted, that part will be deemed to be deleted, and the rest of the section will continue in effect.

Law and jurisdiction

This disclaimer will be governed by and construed in accordance with Swiss law, and any disputes relating to this disclaimer will be subject to the exclusive jurisdiction of the courts of Switzerland.

Contents

Preface

Tired of concealing your overhang fat under layers of your clothes? You are not the only one. Around 33% of American adults are overweight. This is the ideal opportunity to change your delicate, out of shape body into the conditioned, attractive physique you had always wanted. Disregard yo-yo diets and simple weight reduction promise that abandon you feeling like a fat disappointment. It is conceivable to have an incline, activity ceasing body you can hardly wait to flaunt. You've discovered the fat reducing insights TV masters don't want you to think about. Get prepared to discard your fat garments for good.

It's essential to know how fat is kept in the body, so you have a comprehension of how to make the body lose it. Your body needs nourishment to obtain the necessary vitality to perform and feed its cells. The calories in nourishment have vitality usually referred to as calories. The more calories the nourishment contains, the more fuel the body can gain from it. To use the foods' vitality, your body should first process the nourishment. The procedure of assimilation causes the body to smolder some old vitality to get the new vitality from the food. The more difficulties encounter in processing the food, the more vitality/calories are burned.

The body's fuel is classified as protein, carbohydrates or fats. This fuel supports the body and keeps the body working. The leftover calories are in the long run saved in the fat cells. Your body utilizes a part of the nourishments fuel for nutrition. The abundance fuel is in the long run saved as fat in the "fat cells" of your body, around the kidneys and liver.

Fat cells are regularly saved in the chest, hips, and waist area. As the cells increase in size, your body obtains a raw look. The body has a predetermined number of fat cells, and there is just so much fat these cells can save. Once the limit is achieved, fat starts to collect in the muscle coating of your arms and thighs, making unattractive, out of shape limbs.

Mystery #1:
EAT FAT REDUCING FOODS

All nourishments can bring about fat creation, yet certain foods really smolder fat. A few foods have minerals or vitamins that raise digestion system and go about as virtual fat terminators. There are negative calorie nourishments with low calories that reduce additional calories amid processing. Different nourishments, even eaten in little amounts, convey a feeling of totality with next to no calories. Adhering to the right entire foods will definitely decrease the fat profile of your body.

By eating these fat reducing nourishments at the perfect time, in the right sum, the body fat profile begins to decrease. Include foods that lower the probability of fat storing in your body for additional help. Here is a rundown of ordinary nourishments that twofold as secret fat reducers.

Poultry

Poultry, for example, chicken has unique resources that expand the body's metabolic rate, helping you melt additional fat away. Chicken is low in fat and starches with a decent protein profile. Proteins require a ton of vitality to process, and more vitality for proteins to be stocked as fat. It is likewise an incredible source of iron, zinc, and niacin. For best results, expel the skin from poultry before eating to keep away abundance fat.

Salmon and Tuna

Salmon and fish are great sources of protein that furnishes the body with solid fats from omega-3 and omega-6 unsaturated fats. Both substantial fish, while fulfilling, are likewise low in calories and unhealthy full fat. Eating salmon emphatically impacts leptin, the hormone in charge of reducing and saving calories. High leptin levels cause the body to stock fat. Salmon and fish decrease leptin, giving your digestion system the help it needs to smolder calories.

Other Lean Protein

Likewise with different proteins, research has demonstrated the thermic impact of protein is the most of all the macronutrients. Protein requires around 30% of its calories for assimilation and processing. Incline proteins likewise smother the ravenousness decreasing the propensity to gorge. In spite of the fact that poultry has a lower fat profile, incline red meats, for example, top round, incline sirloin, game, and other white meats have a spot in a fat smoldering diet

Citrus Fruits

Citrus fruit climbs up the digestion system while supplying a major measurement of vitamin C, a compound utilized as a part of the procedure of fat burning. Citrus fruits are positioned as the best fat smoldering nourishments you can eat. Oranges, grapefruit, apples and even tomatoes offer these fat reducing qualities. With the extensive assortment, blend a few varieties for various flavors and taste. Citrus fruit viably smolders fat around the hips and waist.

Apples

An apple a day helps in keeping the fat away. Apples contain a substance called pectin that confines the cells from absorbing fat and helps water ingestion from food. This likewise pushes fat stores from the body. The cell reinforcements in apples might likewise decrease overabundance belly fat from a metabolic disorder. Apples have a large quantity of solvent fiber that helps you control hunger torment.

Berries

Strawberries, blueberries, raspberries, blackberries, fruits – take your pick. Fruits, in general, are packed with vitamins and minerals. They are minute on calories and high in water contrasted with refined food. Phenomenal sources of fiber, berries help the digestion system, processing nourishment, and fats. Actually sweet and tasty, a handful of berries will keep you feeling more full and eliminate with the yearning for sugary glasses of artificially enhanced, void calories.

Oatmeal

A huge part of the oats calorie profile is dissolvable fiber. Solvent fiber controls glucose and helps you feel more full. Cereal additionally reduces the danger of coronary illness and reducing cholesterol. Pick antiquated or steel cut oats and eat with fresh fruits. Make a point to screen your serving sizes amid diet stages precisely.

Vegetables

Most vegetables (aside from potatoes, yams, and sweet potatoes) keep up low calories, yet contain vital vitamins and minerals that enhance the body's digestion system. Veggies, for example, spinach, broccoli, cabbage, carrots, and artichokes contain no fat and low starch levels. Indeed, they help in fat smoldering since your body utilizes a larger number of calories to process vegetables than they create. The additional calories expected to process nourishment are taken from body fat reserves. For instance, one serving of

Brussels sprouts has 50 calories, yet the body needs 75 calories to process. That is 25 calories of body fat reduced only for eat your Brussels grows.

Beans

Beans are not just full with minerals; they are likewise low in calories and rich in amino acids. The amino acids in lentils diminish body fat while aids in building muscles, and keep up stable glucose. Likewise, they are fantastic sources of dietary fiber keeping you satisfied longer, decreasing the inclination to gorge.

Eggs

Eggs, a standout amongst the most supplement foods, are a natural superfood.

Their large amounts of protein rev up the digestion system and help you reduce fat. Eggs are hands down one of the best fat reducing nourishments. Among other protein nourishments, eggs have the most bounteous blend of vital amino acids. In spite of having low calories, they are packed with vitamin D, vitamin B12, choline, and selenium. It's been demonstrated eggs don't add to terrible cholesterol, yet improves the great cholesterol required for a sound body. Eggs have every one of the nutrients urgent for good health.

Almonds and Walnuts

Almond and walnuts are an incredible source of healthy fats required for the smooth working of the body's cell structure. Only an ounce of almonds has 12% of the everyday protein stipend and contains calcium and folic corrosive. In addition, the type of vitamin E in walnuts is particularly useful. A handful of nuts is a divine, crunchy snack to fulfill your hunger torments.

Pine Nuts

According to scientists, pine nuts contain a plenitude of healthy unsaturated fats. These unsaturated fats aids eliminate fat amassing in the abdominals. Pine nuts likewise build satiety level hormones alongside the advantages of fat decrease.

SECRET #2:
ADD FAT BOOSTERS TO YOUR DIET

Eating the right nourishment will kick your digestion system into high apparatus and help you reduce undesirable fat. Join fat smoldering nourishments with these fat sponsors to push your digestion system into overdrive.

Mustard

Minor mustard seeds are packed with nutrition including the amino acid tryptophan, omega 3 unsaturated fats, selenium, phosphorus, manganese, magnesium, calcium, iron, niacin, and zinc. They even have a touch of protein and fiber.

The fiery Asian and Mexican assortments briefly accelerate the digestion system like ephedrine fat loss support.

Onions

Onions are fragrant, flavorful and low in calories. In any case, onions can likewise help in weight reduction. They are a source of a nutrient called chromium. Chromium is said to enhance insulin and keep up stable glucose. Along these lines, onions stop glucose crashes and the subsequent instance of the munchies.

Coconut Oil

Coconuts support the body's vitality. Not like margarine or shortening, coconut oil is full of medium chain unsaturated fats utilized as a quick supply of fuel. Use coconut oil in your cooking to speed digestion system, enhance thyroid working and open up fat smoldering.

Hot Peppers

The chemicals that give hot peppers their zest securely speeds up the heart rate. A few individuals can reduce up to 1,000 more calories consistently from eating peppers. Spicy nourishments like chilies and peppers trigger your body to smolder fat. For their flavor and fat smoldering properties, hot peppers are one of the best diet foods.

Green Tea

Green tea altogether diminishes total fat in the waist and skin ranges. Green tea has the catechins, demonstrated to raise your resting metabolic rate. That implies you continue smoldering fat longer, transforming the body into an all around oiled fat reducing machine. It has additionally been demonstrated, the catechins connect with the caffeine in green tea. An immaculate substitute for espresso, green tea is high in preventive agents making it a characteristic invigorate.

SECRET #3
INCREASE WATER INTAKE

Drinking more water offers the body some assistance with reducing fat stores. The kidneys don't work accurately without enough water consumption. If they don't work appropriately, a portion of the heap is discarded to the liver. In the event that the liver is doing the kidney's work, it can't focus on its fundamental employment of metabolizing fat. More fat will stay in the body and fat reducing stops. So drink the appropriate measure of water enhances digestion system and keeps your fat reducing at full limit. Water additionally flushes out poisons and enhances the body's capacity to stay sound.

SECRET#4
BUILD MUSCLES

Muscle keeps you digestion system dynamic and smoldering calories. Adding muscle enhances your body fat ratio composition ratios. Muscles are a dynamic tissue that constantly restores itself so it generally needs calories. While typical cardio smolders fat just amid the activity, weight preparing assembles muscle guaranteeing body fat continues to reduce for throughout the day. The principle source of vitality for muscles is fat. Thus, notwithstanding when unwinding or resting, you keep on smoldering calories. The more bulk on your edge the more beneficial outcome on your digestion system. To avoid your digestion system from getting slow and packing on fat, it is imperative to do weight safe activities to manufacture muscle.

CONCLUSION

Presently you have the secrets to a lovely conditioned body in the palm of your hands. The main thing hindering an incline attractive physical makeup is you. Receive these fat reducing insights into your way of life and you will get results in a matter of weeks. The right diet arrangement will demonstrate to your proper methodologies to join the fat reducing foods to keep your body melting away the fat. There are endless delicious recipes to make the switch easy. Include a weight lifting exercise administration and you will shape your body into an object of craving. Try not to let one more day pass. The new you is prepared to emerge